Living
in a
Cloud
of
SMOKE

Living
in a
Cloud
of
SMOKE

RON DAVIS

authorHOUSE®

AuthorHouse™
1663 Liberty Drive
Bloomington, IN 47403
www.authorhouse.com
Phone: 1-800-839-8640

Published by AuthorHouse   10/22/2012

ISBN: 978-1-4772-5676-3 (sc)
ISBN: 978-1-4772-5677-0 (e)

Library of Congress Control Number: 2012917141

Contents

———➤●◄———

Acknowledgment ix

Introduction xi

The End of a Fifty-Year Seed 1

Let the Twenty-Four Month Battle Begin 11

Living Twenty-Four Hours a Day on Oxygen 17

The Business Decision of a Lifetime 23

Transplant Locations Aren't Limited 33

Up, Up, and Away 39

We're Moving on Up 45

God's Plan Is at Hand 53

The Beginning of the End 61

Strangers in the Night 65

Closing Comments 79

About the Author 95

To my beloved wife, Shawnee, who has been by my side for twenty-two wonderful years. Though at times everything seemed impossible—not knowing for hours, days, and even months what the outcome would be—she was always there. She has been courageous, encouraging, supportive, and, most importantly, loving, helping me through my situation.

In her times alone, tears would fall from her face—tears that touched the very heart of God. Even though I went through a lot over a span of almost two years, so did she. Many times she called out to God, and He heard her cry. He dried her tears; only He knows how.

God blessed me with a helpmate that is unselfish, caring, and giving. She demonstrates the traits, the actions, and the love of God.

Sweetheart, thanks for allowing me to be a part of your life. Thanks for being by my side when I needed it.

Acknowledgment

I would like to give special recognition to a dear friend of mine who is a real inspiration. Time and time again, he has come by to lend a helping hand with this book, assisting with formatting, printing, and computer problems that I encountered while working on my manuscript. Paul Jackson, thanks for all your help, assistance, and brotherly love over the past few years. Each time I have a problem, I can count on you to come by and help. Thanks again, Paul. You are a true friend.

Introduction

This book takes you through a period of my life when I developed a lung disease known as chronic obstructive pulmonary dysfunction disease (COPD), or obstructed air passages. This disease is treated with inhalers, which helps to open the air passages. The only potential long-term cure is through surgery or transplant.

After several months, my diagnosis was changed to severe emphysema. This book takes you through my struggles with that disease, my wait for a new lung, and the miracle of transplant surgery.

You will experience the trials and difficulties I endured before and after surgery. Complications came during my year and a half of dealing with the illness and the surgery—as did miracles and blessings.

The end of the book reflects on events that have taken place since my lung transplant and on how God has blessed me with many opportunities to share what a mighty and loving God we have.

The End of a Fifty-Year Seed

———▸●◂———

Be not deceived, God is not mocked for whatsoever a man soweth, that shall he also reap. (Galatians 6:7)

Some fifty years ago, at eighteen months of age, I hung on Mom's neck while she sewed. I sucked my thumb and had two fingers tucked inside an empty cigarette pack as I breathed the smell of tobacco. Doing so, I planted a seed that led me to become a full-blown, addicted smoker.

Smoking an average of three packs of cigarettes a day for twenty-five years takes its toll. Most smokers will tell you that grabbing a cigarette helps curb nervousness. The only time I truly enjoyed a cigarette was after eating a meal. All the other times were due to the addiction and habitual practice of lighting up every twenty minutes or so to get that "fix" or what most smokers believe is a calmness or soothing. Smoking is no different from abusing any other drug. Once you are addicted, you'll continue to follow the course to satisfy your addiction by any means. In most cases, this addiction ends up destroying not only the life of the addicted person but also the lives of others, including entire families.

Over the years, I found myself trapped in what seemed to be a glass bubble filled with smoke and a smell I could not relinquish. I tried hundreds of times to give up the "habit." I wish I knew the number of times I threw complete packs of cigarettes away, vowing never to smoke again—only to find myself lighting up another smoke within minutes. Once, I wrapped up a pack of cigarettes in a box, tied a bow on top, and placed it in a four-way intersection, hoping someone would pick it up and receive my habit. This was definitely a form of witchcraft, though I didn't think about it at the time.

How stupid I was. I was so addicted, I was willing to do anything to get delivered or else stop smoking. A lot of people that are addicted to alcohol, drugs, sex, or other things end up on a course of destruction. Sometimes it not only costs them their lives but also the lives of others. Just think of the times when addiction to alcohol, drugs, and even careless smoking has caused death or destruction.

The only way to escape from any form of addiction in life is, first, to realize that you are addicted. Second, you must want help. And last, you must realize that you can't do it by yourself. After years of trying to give up the habit, I came to the conclusion that, by myself,

I would never be able to win the battle I was in. It seemed that all the prayers I had prayed over the years were in vain. I knew that God wanted me to be free from tobacco. Yet I could not understand why I could not just lay them down and walk away from them.

God tells us in His Word that our body is the temple of God. Knowing this, we should understand that God will not possess or take up residence in a temple that is not clean or pure. Now, don't take me wrong; I'm not saying a person has to "get cleaned up," before coming to God. There is no way we could ever get clean enough to invite Jesus in our life. This is why He tells us to come as we are. Many people let Satan convince them that they are not good enough to live the Christian life or that they must first give up their habits or stop practicing their sinful ways before God will accept them.

This thought from Satan is totally false and straight from the pit of hell, so don't listen to him. God can work only in those willing to take him at His Word, to trust Him to take charge of their life, and to allow Him to bring change in it. God loves the sinner but not the sin. As a matter of a fact, He can't even look on sin. But He does look on the sinner whom He loves and desires to fellowship with. He cannot fellowship with us until we invite Him into our life.

Being free from a life of addiction, whether it is alcohol, drugs, tobacco, lust, or any type of sin, can only come about by yielding ourselves over to the One that can bring everlasting deliverance. That one is Jesus. He requires us to trust Him, take him at His Word, and allow Him to change us.

The reason many fail is because we expect instant change. Sometimes change comes that way, but for most it happens over a period of trusting and obeying. As the old hymn says, "trust and obey, for there's no other way to be happy in Jesus, but to trust and obey."

Another way we can receive deliverance and freedom from addictions is to begin speaking positive. Speak the results you want rather than the problem you are facing. In doing so, you turn faith into reality. The solution rather than the problem. As long as we speak defeat and despair, we will never conquer the battles we are facing. This is why addicted people often fall back into their addiction; they allow negative thoughts to control their thinking. Once a person quits saying "can't," they *can* do anything. They have to learn to replace old, defeating, negative thoughts with positive, conquering thoughts.

In the summer of 1992, as my wife, Shawnee, and I planned our vacation, I decided the time had come for me to give up smoking "once and for all." I was sick and tired of cigarettes controlling my life. (That's what it is—control. The addiction is a control, of your situation.) A couple months before going on vacation, I began to tell everyone, "Come vacation, I am giving up smoking." But they probably thought otherwise, because I just kept on puffing, as usual.

One day a small voice inside me said, "Give your cigarette money away."

I thought, *What?*

Again, I heard, "Give your cigarette money away."

Dwelling, on what I had heard, I thought, *What do I have to lose? I've tried everything else.* For the next six weeks up until we were ready to leave, I did not know when or how I was to give away my cigarette money. We were to travel out on Friday, August 25, headed for Wisconsin. On the twenty-fourth I heard that voice again rise within me, saying, "Give our cigarette money [the amount I normally spent for two weeks] to the guy that works with you." So I did.

As we left for vacation the next evening, I prayed a little prayer, thanking God for delivering me from smoking. From that moment on, I have not smoked another cigarette.

While we were in Wisconsin, it seemed that everyone I was around smoked. But I never desired a cigarette. The smell that once caused me to want to smoke had no effect on me. I definitely knew this time was different than all the other times I had tried to quite. Why? Because I had finally tapped in to the Deliverer. Once I recognized my deliverance was from Jesus and not from my own ability; I was able to receive my deliverance.

If you need deliverance from any situation, ask God to set you free from whatever is keeping you from living in the liberty and freedom Jesus desires you live. His Word declares, "Beloved I wish above all things that thou mayest prosper and be in health, even as thy soul prospereth" (3 John 2). God desires the best for us and longs to share it with us. Yet He will not force Himself on us. He is standing near to come into our life. It is up to us to give Him an invitation.

Once we invite Him, we have new meaning and purpose. Instead of living for our own desires, we begin to try to please Him and others around us. The greatest thing of all is, once our life has ended here, we begin a life of eternity with Him. He has promised this to those who are his children.

There is no reason on earth we should allow anything or anyone to have control over us. Nothing should prevent us from living in total victory. Total victory comes once we place our life in the hand of God.

Let's move on to look at the huge battle I fought from 1997 to 1999. Though those twenty-four months were trying, I'm glad I didn't have to face it alone. I had God to lead me through it. I also had an understanding wife, family, and friends, which made it a lot easier. Whenever we have God on our side, we are bound to win.

Let the Twenty-Four Month Battle Begin

———⟫•⟪———

*Be not afraid nor dismayed by
reason of this great multitude;
for the battle is not yours but God's.
(2 Chronicles 20:15)*

It was the first weekend of December, 1997. Mom had some items she needed to be picked up at my sister Karen's home in Fort Walton Beach, Florida. Shawnee and I agreed to fly down, rent a truck, load it up, and return home the following morning. This was my first indication that my breathing was becoming difficult.

I had just finished working on a project in Atlanta the previous year. For nearly nine months, I had traveled back and forth from Asheville to Atlanta for work. I was blessed to work for some friends of mine, Jimmy and Joann Thompson. They owned and operated several Christian television broadcast stations in South Carolina. Their home station is TV 16 (Dove Broadcasting) out of Greenville, South Carolina. In the spring of 1996, they started operating TV 57, off I-85 in Atlanta. The entire area was preparing for the Summer Olympics.

Joann was having difficulty finding someone to help her fulfill a lifelong dream and vision God had given her of opening a station in the Atlanta area. A friend of mine approached me to consider going down to see if I might be able to help with remodeling her new TV station. After several weeks of thinking and praying about it, I decided to give it a try.

I had thought I would only be commuting back and forth for six to eight weeks, but one knows how that is when remodeling is involved. I would drive down on Sunday evenings and check into the motel less than a mile from the station. The next morning, I'd grab a quick breakfast before starting work. Every few days, Joann would come up with a new project or different idea—often something that seemed impossible. Every time, her impossible ideas came along (and she had a barrel full of them), I knew I would spend extra time praying, asking the Master Builder (Jesus) to assist me.

Thank God, we were in one accord. Of course, things always turns out exactly the way they are meant, being God was involved. I enjoyed the work and the challenges I faced while working there. God taught me a lot and conditioned me for things to come.

On Thursday afternoons, I would drive back home to tend to business before returning again on Sunday. As I worked and traveled all those months, I never noticed much difficulty in breathing. I was still able to lift heavy objects, walk steep grades, and do almost anything I wanted.

It wasn't until the following year that I really began to notice my breathing difficulties. I began feeling tired all the time. In December, as I returned from my sister's in the rental truck, I realized something had to be done.

After persuasion by wife and mom, I made an appointment with a pulmonary doctor to see why I was having shortness of breath. My symptoms were the same as my brother Ray's, who had gone through a heart triple bypass. My test results concluded that I had chronic obstructive pulmonary dysfunction disease (COPD), or obstructed air passage.

I was prescribed several inhalers, and over the next several months, I continued working as usual. At times I would get short of breath and exhausted from walking up steps or steep inclines. I would take a couple of puffs on my inhaler just to have enough strength to finish working. Many days I would barely make it home.

Each day brought increasing pain. At one point, I decided to get a second opinion concerning my health. Things were not getting any better; day-to-day living was an increasing struggle. Living normally like was a thing of the past.

I started looking for a pulmonary group covered by our insurance company. In Hendersonville, North Carolina, I came across Western North Carolina Pulmonary. My first office visit was in September 1998 to see a pulmonary physician, Dr. Ward. I was very impressed by the way he took extensive time to explain my problem and personal concerns and solutions. I was assured that God had sent me to the right place.

Upon leaving my examining room, Dr. Ward remarked, "Brother, I'll be praying for you." The door closed, and immediately I heard a little tap on the door. Dr. Ward came back in and sat down beside me. "Brother, I don't need to pray for you," he said. "I need to pray *with* you." How astonished I was to have a doctor be willing to take time to pray with me. Seldom does anyone take time to pray, especially in the world we live today.

Every one of my visits with Dr. Ward ended with him praying for God's will and healing for my body, and my prayer of God's blessing and direction in his life, family and practice. The entire staff at WNC Pulmonary was great; they made you feel relaxed.

I've come to discover that, no matter what situation we face, God has a purpose and plan that places us in "perfect peace," even in the midst of calamity.

Living Twenty-Four
Hours a Day
on Oxygen

————➤●◄————

*Behold I will cause breath to
enter into you and ye shall live.
(Ezekiel 37:5)*

―――⫸●⫷―――

By mid-October 1998, my doctor requested that I be on oxygen twenty-four hours a day. His diagnosis was severe emphysema. Struggling to breath, I was using my inhalers several times throughout the day. Picking up large items or walking any distance would completely take away my breath. I would have to stand and rest before continuing with whatever, I was doing. The only relief I could get was when I used my inhalers.

One day when I was on oxygen, I needed to enlarge the opening for a new oven. I expected it to be an hour-long job, but it took almost three hours. As I worked, I really struggled. It was difficult to breath and move while hooked up to oxygen; the line was long and constantly getting in the way. By the time I finished, it was 12:25, and I was exhausted. But I had an appointment for pulmonary rehabilitation at one in Hendersonville, the next town over, thirty miles away. Being in a hurry, I became frustrated, and my breathing became more labored. By the time I arrived home, my breathing was really awful.

I hurried inside, changed my clothes—and out the door I went. It's about a fifteen-minute drive to the hospital, and it was almost one. I arrived about ten minutes late, parked the car, and rushed inside. I was totally beside myself. You would have thought I had been in a fight.

My pulmonary instructor noticed my color wasn't right, so she had me sit down and rest. After taking my oxygen level count, she saw that my oxygen level was unstable, so she called Dr. Ward. He suggested I stop by. I drove around the block to the doctor's office. Feeling dizzy from my low oxygen levels, I ran over the curb, pulled out in front of another car, and almost knocked down the handicap sign as I parked at the doctor's office. It's a wonder I didn't kill someone or cause an accident. I was really out of touch and didn't even know it.

In the office, the nurses rushed me to one of the examination rooms and put me on oxygen. Within a few minutes, the doctor came in. After my examination, I was admitted to the hospital, as my oxygen level remained unstable. When I remained still and lying down, I was okay. Whenever I stood up or moved around, my oxygen level would hit rock bottom. Over the next several days, the doctor ordered numerous tests to determine what was going on with my body. Eventually, the right medicines were prescribed to help stabilize my oxygen levels.

The Business Decision of a Lifetime

For the day of the Lord is near in the valley of decision.

(Joel 3:14)

———⟫●⟨———

Once I was admitted to the hospital, my mind started racing for answers of what would become of my ability to work, my business, my bills. *What about this? What about that?* I was really mixed up, nervous, and full of fear. The only thing I could do was what most of us do: have a pity party. Boy! Did I ever have one! I cried and cried till I could not cry any longer. After a while, I started again.

Friday morning, January 15th, I woke up and began crying out to God to help me with all I was facing. At that moment, I was worried that I would not be able to continue my reputation as a respected businessman after twenty years of service to the community and keep providing service to companies that I represented and installed for. Immediately, a friend's name came to mind. I picked up the phone, gave him a call, and worked out an arrangement for him to handle upcoming installations. Next I talked to God and reminded Him that I had given Him the business years ago, and I was only operating it as He gave me the ability.

I said, "Lord this is your business, and I appreciate you allowing me to operate all these years. Now may be the time for me to step down and give it up, if I must. I really want to keep it, but I realize if I have to give it up, I will. Your will in my life is more important than my business—or anything else "After talking to God, I thought everything would be all right, but it wasn't. I started balling again. I cried and cried and kept on crying. I cried till I could cry no more.

Then, all of a sudden, a peace came over me as I heard a small voice inside say, "Ron, it's okay. Everything is going to be taken care of. I'm going to bring forth something new and place within you a ministry where you can spread the good news of deliverance, healing, and freedom to a hurting world."

That evening my son Geoff, who lived in Houston, called to see how I was doing. We started discussing whether or not he had found a church to attend. He said he planned on going somewhere soon. My reply was, "Son, let me tell you like Jesus told Judas at the Last Supper: 'Whatever you do, do it quickly.' "I love you and want to see you and your family in heaven, but if you're not there, I won't miss you." Once in heaven, our heart will be focused on heavenly surroundings.

Things—including friends and family—on earth will not affect us like they do now. Though we love our families and want to see them saved, should they not be in heaven, it will not have any effect on our thinking. Heaven is a place where we will only be able to think on "heavenly things." If that weren't the case, our minds would not be transformed like God says He will do when Christ returns to take us home (1 Corinthians 15:48-49).

That night I woke up around midnight. I lay there tossing back and forth, trying to go back to sleep. The room was dark, except for a small amount of light from the bathroom. Lying on my back, I dozed for maybe fifteen to twenty minutes. For some strange reason, I woke up and focused on the heat vent above my bed. I noticed what appeared to be a black cloud hovering right in front of the vent. I closed my eyes. When I looked again to be sure I wasn't dreaming, the black cloud seemed to sway back and forth.

All of a sudden I began to have an eerie feeling. Thoughts began going through my mind. A voice within me said, "You're going down. You're going to lose everything you own. Your wife is going to become a widow." These thoughts kept coming to me.

The only thing I knew to do was to pray. I cried out to God asking for divine protection. Even as I was praying, Satan said, "I'm here to take you out." I continued to pray and trust God and His word. After a moment, I opened my eyes and focused on the vent.

The black cloud was still there, but there was a second cloud in front of the black cloud. This cloud was white. As I continued focusing on both clouds, a peace began to flow inside me. Then a small voice said, "Ron, I've placed My cloud in front of Satan's cloud. He cannot come through the blood."

"Praise God!" I shouted. I not only *felt* God's peace and protection, I also was able to *see* it. Lying there, full of God's presence, I fell asleep. Later I awoke again. I looked to see if the clouds were still there, but they were gone. Still bubbling with the peace of God, I lay there praising and thanking Him for His protection.

A couple days later, Geoff called again and told me about some problems he and his wife had been having. They had decided to separate. He said they had jumped into the marriage and realized it was a mistake. Geoff had been running from God, yet I knew that, for the first time in several years, God was doing a work of restoration.

Geoff asked if I would give him a chance to operate the business. My reply was "Of course you can." I explained to Geoff that I was willing to give him a try. He said that his plans were to be home around the middle of February, and he would start training then to take over the business. I told him that if he would allow God to enter our relationship as a business partner, he would have nothing to worry about.

So in mid-February 1999, Geoff and his son, Andrew, moved back to Asheville. They moved in with his mom. His original plan was to work a while and then move behind his mom in a mobile home. At the time, he was struggling financially and didn't know how to fix the problem. You know, we've all been there at one time or another. With his back against the wall, he committed himself to God and stood his ground, refusing to let Satan destroy his life.

Within a few short weeks, things started coming together. Geoff was able to save well over two thousand dollars on his auto insurance. He was also able to purchase a new manufactured home. And God even reserved a single private lot that was left "vacant" (it should have been rented within hours) close to his church and Andrew's school.

Geoff started working the business, installing appliances,and doing minor repairs. Because I could not physically do the work, I instructed him on what needed to be done. I would only have to instruct him once. He performed exceedingly well, beyond my expectations. Plans are for him to take over the business in the near future.

On my last day at the hospital, the doctor made arrangements for me to travel to Duke University Hospital. He felt my situation had become too severe, and Duke was more capable of diagnosing my illness. On Saturday, March 13, we drove to Winston-Salem and spent the weekend with my Aunt Lois. On Sunday afternoon, we continued on to Duke. The trip was about an hour and half from Winston-Salem. Shawnee and I checked into a motel about two miles from the hospital.

Early Monday morning, after extensive testing, the lung transplant surgeon told me that normally one option was to have a lung reduction in which they would cut out the bad parts of the lung and save the good tissue. But in my case the damage was too severe, so a reduction was out. The only other option was a lung transplant. At that time, our insurance covered only lung reduction at Duke. So we were a dead end. Even though we were discouraged, we still had confidence that God would bring us through. We continued to acknowledge that God was in control.

We drove back to Winston-Salem, spent the night, and drove back home on Tuesday afternoon. The hardest thing about the trip was having my wife lug all that oxygen around. I was using the CO_2 cylinders for outside use and a roll-about concentrator for home use. We ended up taking eight or nine cylinders with us for the weekend. She also had to carry my nebulizer—a machine used to help open my air passages.

To use the nebulizer, I would place medicine in the mouthpiece and breathe into it for ten to twenty minutes until all the medicine was gone. I had to do this four times a day, in addition to my other medicines. It took a while to get used to taking all the medicines and doing the breathing treatments, but eventually it became routine. Being attached to a fifty-foot oxygen line took some time getting used to also, but after a while it wasn't too bad either. I learned to accept it. When you know that it is only temporal, you can cope with it a lot easier.

A week or two after returning from Duke, plans were in the making to locate to a suitable medical facility for a lung transplant. Working with our insurance company, I was introduced to Deborah, a lung transplant coordinator for North Carolina. Over the months to follow, Deborah and I became close friends, although we never met. After speaking to her the first time, I knew she was special; I felt as if I had known her for years. She had a sweet, understanding spirit. Each time I called Deborah, she would encourage me with the words she spoke. Her faith touched me each time we spoke. It is very uplifting to know God places people all around you whenever you need assurance that everything is going to be all right. Time and time again, He did that for me, reminding me that He loves me and is concerned for my well-being.

Transplant Locations Aren't Limited

———⟫•⟪———

For thou art my rock and fortress;
therefore for thy name's sake
lead me, and guide me.
(Psalm 31:3)

Weeks after returning from Duke, we received a call informing us that there were several medical facilities throughout the United States that could perform a lung transplant and take my medical insurance. After prayerful consideration, we chose the University of Wisconsin Hospital in Madison. The university was listed as one of the nation's leading facilities in lung and heart transplants. We also found out that the surgeon, Dr. Love, had a 100 percent success rate in performing lung transplants. Also, my wife's family lived within an hour or so of the hospital. We were informed that anytime someone receives a transplant, it is very important that they have as much support as possible.

After our initial contact with UW Hospital, we were instructed to have the medical records from my pulmonary doctor's office and those from Duke

University forwarded to UW for review. A few weeks later, we received word that I had been turned down because my lungs were not bad enough to be transplanted. Can you imagine receiving a report like that after praying and believing that God was restoring your health? I thought, *I'm not going to accept this.* Then this thought came to my mind: *Whose report will you believe? I shall believe the report of the Lord.*

When we put our trust in the Lord, we don't have to accept a bad report. Our God is bigger than the worst report we could ever receive. If we accept every bad report that comes along, we will never have any victory. Everyone would fail, give up, or die without ever receiving healing or victory. Going to doctors and taking medicines would be useless. I am speaking of the medical field, but this is true of every situation we face. Things may look bad at times, and your world may look as though it's falling apart, but it doesn't have to end up that way.

The world, and especially Satan, would have you believe that this is the way things have to be. It is for a lot people, but it doesn't have to be. God wants us to believe in Him and in the promises of His Word. He wants us to "prosper and be in health, even as [our] soul prospers." Putting our trust in God causes supernatural results that cannot be explained. That's why it's called a "miracle."

And this is what happened: Neither of my doctors accepted the decision we had received. Within days, both contacted UW Hospital and persuaded them to take a look at me in person. On paper, I did not look as sick as I was in person.

Within a week, an appointment was set for me to be examined. We flew up in the middle of May, and I completed all the necessary tests. After returning home, we waited patiently, hoping to receive the call that I would be on the transplant list. Praise God! On June 1, Debbie, my transplant coordinator at UW, called to inform me that I was officially on the list. Soon I received a pager so Debbie could page me when a lung come available and tell me what procedures to take. From June to mid-September, we waited anxiously for a call.

In August, we traveled to Madison for an annual transplant picnic on a Sunday afternoon. Our family was the largest in attendance. We enjoyed the afternoon as we met transplant recipients, their family members, and the transplant team. And the food was great too. Many people we were introduced to provided vital information concerning the transplant surgery and the support needed after surgery. We received tons of medical information too.

Later that evening, at the motel, we had felt good knowing what we had learned about transplants about what would help us after my transplant. After a couple of days visiting the family and a clinic appointment, we flew back home.

Up, Up, and Away

And he rode upon a cherub,
and did fly; yea he did fly
upon the wings of the wind.
(Psalm 18:10)

———⟫●⟪———

After returning from church on Sunday, September 19, 1999, and eating lunch, I was thinking of resting for an hour or so, when the phone rang.(I was surprised, for I thought they would have paged me.) On the other end, the caller said," Are you ready for your lung?"

I replied, "Sure, who is this?" (I thought someone was pulling a joke on me). "Are you serious?"

She replied, "Yes, I'm serious. Don't eat or drink anything. We're calling Air Medical and will call you back shortly to let you know what time to be at the airport."

For the most part, we were packed and ready to leave. But when the call came, I went blank. I couldn't think straight. I tried to think of everything I needed to do, but I was five miles and two hours ahead of my brain. Thank God, we took time to pray. And everything got taken care of.

My brother Julian came over and took us to the jet port. As we arrived, the medical jet had already landed and was refueling. By 4:15 p.m., we were in the air. You've heard the saying, "A great day for flying." It was. The sky was so blue, sprinkled with a cloud every so often—a beautiful fall afternoon. The flight was smooth and fast, and there were only five of us aboard: Shawnee, me, a nurse, the pilot, and the co-pilot. Our flight time was just over three and half hours.

As we approached the southwest corner of Michigan and Wisconsin, we could see thick clouds forming ahead of us. Looking out the window, Shawnee pointed to one huge black cloud in the distance to east of us. As I looked, we turned to each other, knowing a rough ride was in store. As we kept watching the cloud's movement, we noticed it rapidly moving in our direction. Among all the clouds in the sky at the time, this one did not fit. It was definitely out of place.

As the pilot turned the plane toward the southwest, down into the thick clouds we went. Nervously holding on, I begin to pray and pray hard. Knowing we were headed right into the middle of those thick clouds and being unable to see the ground below made me uptight. After four or five minutes that seemed to be eternity, I looked out the front of the plane and could see the ground. Within minutes we were lined up with the runway and ready to land. The pilot dropped the landing gear, and soon we were on the ground and taxing to the terminal.

An ambulance was waiting at the Madison Airport, ready to transport me to the hospital. As we left the airport, the ambulance driver turned the siren on and started hustling through the traffic. It took about fifteen minutes to get to the hospital. As we approached the emergency entrance, Shawnee's family was waiting for us.

The hospital attendants placed me on a bed and rolled me to my room. By seven, Central Time, I was prepped and ready for surgery.

I was scheduled to receive the left lung only. The right lung was for a patient already in surgery. The nurse kept coming by, giving me updates as to when I would be going to the operating room. Every hour or so, she would say that there was delay due to difficulties they were experiencing with the other surgery. Around 1:30 a.m., we were informed that the other lung patient's left lung was reacting to his new right lung. The doctor had to make a decision as to what to do. He decided to replace the left lung, too, to save the patient's life.

We felt the doctor made the right decision, and the lung was not meant for me. Our main concern at the moment was that the patient would pull through surgery. We began to intercede on his behalf, asking God's healing power to touch him.

Early the next morning, the doctor stopped by my room. He explained that he had no choice but to do what he did. I assured him I was okay with that, saying, "The lung was not for me." I really felt good about it and was glad that the patient came through the transplant successfully.

We're Moving
on Up

———❥❦❧———

*The steps of a good man are
ordered by the Lord.
(Psalm 37:23)*

My doctor suggested we relocate to the Madison area because of the amount time it took for us to arrive by air. Though it was only three and half hours, including the time change, he thought it was cutting it close, particularly with my blood pressure being excessively high. Note: When a hospital team goes out to harvest transplant organs, there are critical timetables, for the time the organs are harvested and re-transplanted in a patient. My travel time from North Carolina to University Hospital, in Madison was also to the max.

We lived out of suitcases until we were able to move into an apartment seven miles from the hospital. It had two bedrooms, a kitchen, a dining room, and a living room. Off of the living room was a private deck with a sliding door. We spent a lot of time sitting around reading, praying, and watching TV. Shawnee worked on several puzzles with little help from me; puzzles are definitely one thing I don't have patience for.

Each time we went out, we had to fill my oxygen tanks, strap them over our shoulders, and carry them everywhere we went. So I could get enough oxygen, we started carrying two tanks each time we went. As I got weaker and weaker, Shawnee had to carry both tanks. Most of the time, she did the shopping alone, because I would be too weak to walk far. When we went somewhere, I often sat in the car while she attended to whatever needed to be done.

Sitting around day after day, week after week, began to take its toll not only on me but also on Shawnee. Each time the phone rang, we jumped to our feet, hoping a lung had been received. We spent time away from the apartment as much as possible. Shopping, going to movies, visiting the family—anything to pass the time away. Though it was inconvenient carrying oxygen around, we felt better getting out of the apartment.

On Wednesday, October 6, Shawnee flew home to North Carolina to get our car and more clothes. When we flew up in September, we had taken only one suitcase. We thought we would be there for only a few weeks, so we had not packed enough clothes. We had no idea we would be there for three and a half months. As the weather began to change, we knew we would definitely need heavier clothing.

My brother-in-law Terry stayed with me while Shawnee was gone. He also had to drive me to rehab therapy. On Friday evening, October 8th Shawnee's sister Jo and her daughters came over to stay with me. Shawnee and her sister Jean with her two sons arrived home around 2:30 a.m. Saturday morning on October the 9th. During their stay, someone commented, "Ron, wouldn't it be nice if you got your lung while they are here."

As we were returning from the grocery store, on Monday, October the 11th, I received a page and was instructed to sit tight and not to eat or drink anything until they got back to us. The call came; the lungs were no good.

The next day we were returning from shopping, walking toward the apartment, when the pager sounded again. I returned the call and was informed that a "set of lungs" was available. Once again, I was instructed not to eat or drink anything until they called back. About an hour passed when the phone rang; I was to come on to the hospital.

Shawnee started collecting everything, including my suitcase, oxygen tanks, medicines, and the baby. Did I say baby? Jean had gone shopping with her sister Jo and had left baby Brody with us. As we loaded the car, we realized we had no car seat. With no time to waste, we decided that we would strap Brody between us, and get going to the hospital. Thank God, we did not get pulled over. It would have been something explaining the situation we were in. We arrived at the hospital around five in the evening. Soon Shawnee's family arrived for moral support.

Her family was so supportive. Never a day passed, without one of them calling to check on me, coming over to visit, or assisting Shawnee. We would have had a difficult time without their help. I know my own family would have done the same, had the transplant been done closer to home.

I was taken to my room and prepped, and then we waited until 11:00 p.m. Then my bed was rolled to the area just outside the operating room. At about 12:15, word was received that the donor's lungs were being harvested ninety miles away, in Rockford, Illinois. However, they were not holding air, due to a tear in the bottom of the lungs. Somehow, while the doctors were harvesting the lungs, the tissue stuck to the ribcage and tore as the lungs were being removed from the body.

The doctor came in and explained the situation, saying that if he had an opportunity to examine the lungs firsthand, he might be able to use them. But by then it may be too late, and he felt it was necessary for him to move on to a heart transplant patient waiting on the operating table. He made me feel good when he said, "There is a right lung out there for you, somewhere."

The doctor told me I could stay the night or go home. I decided to leave. When Shawnee's mom returned to the hospital with my clothes and oxygen, we decided to go out for breakfast. After all, I was starved. I had not eaten for ten hours. Maybe longer.

We went to a nearby Perkins restaurant and ordered breakfast. It was after three in the morning by the time we got home and into bed. On Friday, October 15, Shawnee rode back to North Carolina with her sister Jean and her sons, Justin and Brody. While home, she completed a continuing education course for her optical license. And on Monday, she flew back to Madison.

God's Plan Is
at Hand

———►●◄———

For it is God which worketh in
you both to will and to do
of his good pleasure.
(Philippians 2:13)

———>◄◄◄———

During the first week of November, Shawnee and I discussed going to church. Thursday of that week, I was praying and talking to God about my healing when God spoke to me and said, "Ron, all healing is divine, whether it comes supernaturally or I decide to use a man [in my case, a surgeon]. All healing is from the Father above" I sat there amazed. I'd known this all my life, but now it registered like never before. After fifty-two years, it was as though a light bulb just came on. I began praising God for this revelation like never before. A little later, I was flipping through the Yellow Pages and came across a Pentecostal church not far from where we were staying.

On Saturday night, November 13, at about 3:00 a.m., I was awakened out of my sleep, shouting, "Yes." While sleeping, I had been in God's presence, and He had called my name. So I had sat up straight in the bed and answered His call. I didn't know at the time what had caused me to shout as I did. I hardly remember waking up or talking in my sleep. But I do remember standing in God's presence; it seemed so real. I don't quite understand what I was saying yes to, other than letting God know I was in agreement with Him. If you think about it, would we really want to answer any other way? Would we really want to say no to Christ?

This happened at the very time some friends back home, Wade and Gwen, were praying. I found out a week later that God had stirred them to get out of bed and to begin praying that my health situation would come to a head. They prayed that I would receive my healing or surgery soon. They began praying at 2:30 and prayed for about an hour and a half—the exact time I sat up and answered yes. What a mighty God we serve! Praise God for the blessings he bestows on us, even when we're unaware of it.

On Sunday morning, we attended church as we had decided. We were warmly welcomed and then entered the sanctuary, where we joined in the praise and worship. The pastor delivered a great message, and afterward he opened the altar for prayer. The woman who had welcomed us came over and asked if we would like to have the church stand with us in prayer. I replied, "Certainly," so we walked to the altar.

Once there, the pastor came over to ask what my request was. I explained to him that I was waiting for a lung transplant and was trusting God for a healing. He immediately had the musicians stop playing and explained my request to the church. He asked for the elders of the church to stand behind Shawnee and me, as a point of contact and prayer support.

The associate pastor anointed my head with oil, and prayer began flowing from every direction. The power of God was all around. We could actually feel a tangible power all over our bodies. God's power was so strong I could hardly stand. I really felt the power and peace of the Holy Spirit.

After the service, our bodies continued to shake and tremble from the awesome power of God. What a great and blessed feeling we experienced!

The very next day—Monday, November 15, we received a phone call after lunch. They had a possible set of lungs. Thinking it might be like the last few calls, we didn't get too excited. (See how our human thinking kicks in—even after we decide to trust God? He answers our prayers, and we still doubt, even when our miracle is front and center.) Around four that afternoon, the phone rang, and I was asked to come to the hospital. Everything looked as if it were a "go." After making a few calls, packing some clothes, and gathering all my medicines, we made our way to the hospital.

I was given a room where I undressed and put on a hospital gown. The nurses came in and prepped me for surgery. I was told I would probably not go down to the OR (operating room) until around nine—a two-hour wait. Shawnee and I waited in the room, talking to pass the time away. Periodically, the nurse would come in to give us an update. At about 9:15 the door swung open, and off we went down the hall to the elevator. They placed me into the holding room, where I waited to be rolled into the operating room to receive my lungs.

I had been scheduled to receive only one lung. But the news now was that I was going to receive both a right and a left lung. The donor (a twenty-two year-old-man who had lost his life in a car accident in Milwaukee) had been on life support until his parents made the decision to donate his organs. I praise God for their unselfish decision to share their son's life that I might live.

In the operating room, the anesthetist placed a mask over my mouth. He informed me he was going to fit the mask and make sure it felt okay. I was about to ask him how long it would be before I fell off to sleep, when I heard a sweet voice, saying, "Hey, baby, it's all over. You're going to be fine." It was the voice of my lovely wife.

The next three days I remained in ICU. On Friday afternoon, I was moved to a step-down room, where I remained for eight days. During that time, Shawnee and my children planned a surprise Thanksgiving visit. With all the medication I was on and with me being so emotional, they were uncertain if I would be able to handle their visit. Two or three days before the visit, the nurses started giving me medication to keep me from being so emotional.

Their arrival certainly was a surprise, and it was definitely a great time to be thankful. Shawnee opened the door and said, "Honey, you've got some visitors." When I saw who was out in the hall, I began to weep uncontrollable. After the shock, they became tears of joy. My daughter, Leslie; with my son-in-law Nathan; my fourteen-month-old grandson, Chase; my son, Geoff; and my ten-year-old grandson, Andrew, had all made the fourteen-hour trip.

The news had spread around the hospital, and it seemed that everyone knew my family was coming up to visit. Everyone except me. It was the best-kept secret. I knew nothing. I usually can detect when something is about to happen, but not this time. I was totally overtaken by surprise. The next three days were filled with a great time of fellowship.

On Saturday night, the kids left for home. I hated to see them leave, but I had been so uplifted by their visit.

Later that evening, I was moved to another room that was much larger. *Too bad I didn't have it while the kids were here,* I thought.

The next day, I began feeling nauseated and dizzy. Whenever I sat on the side of my bed, I would gag and begin to throw up. And when I ate, I'd end up either gagging or throwing up all I had eaten. The gagging was caused by some of the medicine I was taking and because my digestive tract was still shut down from the surgery. This condition continued for four to five days, making me miserably sick.

I continued to pray that God would deliver me from this sickness. A voice inside me arose and said, "Everyone's prayers have been focused on the transplant; now prayer needs to be in the area of the stomach and digestive tract." I turned to Shawnee and asked her to call our friend back home, Ray Curtis. We asked him to have our church family pray for the area the Lord had spoken to me about. Within minutes, I felt a peace come over me and the assurance that I was on the right track to recovery. Though I continued to be sick as before, over the next several days, I knew deliverance was on the way.

The Beginning of the End

———⮞●⮜———

For I know, the thoughts I think

toward you, saith the Lord,

thoughts of peace and not of evil,

to give you an expected end.

(Jeremiah 29:10)

It was approaching the midnight hour of November 30 when I awoke and focused my eyes on six to eight black, wavy objects hovering right above my bed. They appeared to be startled that I had noticed them. To make sure I wasn't dreaming, I blinked once or twice, took another look, and then they disappeared. Very tired and sleepy, I fell back to sleep.

I awoke again at 2:30 a.m. As I thought about what had occurred earlier, I began to call on God, asking that His protection and healing would flow throughout my room. Soon I was asleep again. At 4:30 I awoke again, needing to use the bathroom. It was also time for my weight check. Each morning the nurse on duty would come by to weigh me. Lying there waiting for her to step in, I fell asleep for the third time. I ended up sleeping three long hours. My dream included an understanding of the objects I had seen earlier.

I have written down a dream I had that night and the interpretation the Lord gave me. I understand that it seems weird; in the natural, it makes no sense at all. After seeing it through the eyes of God, you will see that God is forever with us.

At times, God may allow dreams to appear so that we dwell on them and get information that is useful in our day-to-day living and walk. God can speak to us at any time or in any way He'd like. He can and may use any source He deems fits to get His message across. God's Word tells us how He spoke through a donkey and even a bush. He also mentioned in His Word that the mountains and rocks will cry praise to Him if we don't. At times, we can hear His voice in the wind, rain, or trees—to name a few. God has His way of getting our attention. Oh, that we might become better listeners.

Strangers in the Night

———⟢⟣———

And a stranger will they not follow,
but will flee from him: for they
know not the voice of strangers.
(John 10:5)

In my dream, I had driven to a store. It was an auto supply store or a mechanic's shop or something similar. I parked the car and then walked toward the town shopping area. As I got closer, I saw that many of the buildings were on fire. Flames were everywhere, high above the buildings. Hugh plate-glass windows shattered, and flames soared out with big balls of black smoke. Power lines and trees were down, and many were blocking the streets. It was total destruction everywhere I looked.

As fear set in, I began to run. I turned a corner and noticed that I was in front of a store that seemed familiar; it was an appliance store that I had done business with for years. The fire was rapidly making its way toward the store; it was just minutes away. As I entered the store, I noticed my friends Bruce and Susie frantically trying to rescue three dogs trapped beneath the floor. They were unable to find an opening in the floor. I explained to Bruce that I could cut a hole large enough for the dogs to escape.

As I began to cut the floor, I found myself beneath the floor in a pool of water along with the dogs. The basement had become flooded to about waist high. All three dogs were struggling to stay alive. I reached out for the first dog and grabbed him. But he slipped out of my hands. Something slick was all over his body—some type of oil or grease. By then, the second dog was swimming beside me, so I reached out and lifted him up to safety through the hole in the floor.

I returned to the middle of the flooded basement, where I found the first dog. Again I reached for him, knowing that I would have to really hold on tight. He began to pull away, and I clutched him a little tighter. Doing so, I was able to lift him up to safety.

As I waded to the far end of the room, I saw the third dog paddling; his head was barely above water. I reached out, and he came toward me as if to say, "Thanks for rescuing me." Afterward, I climbed to safety.

Coming out of the store basement, I beheld the most beautiful mountain scene I have ever laid my eyes on. I was totally overtaken by its beauty. Every inch of the mountain was laid out with breathtaking artwork, such as rainbow-colored flowers, bushes, and shrubs. Rocks shimmered and sparkled as the sun's rays beamed down from above. Precious gems and jewels were embedded throughout the entire area.

Walking along, I noticed a couple of friends of mine. Though there was fire, flooding, hurricane winds, and total destruction all around, this one place was calm and peaceful. As I called out their names, it was as though they didn't hear. I ran up to them and tried my best to have them turn and look at the mountain. But they pulled away, their minds preoccupied with the destruction in front of them.

As I continued to make my way through the streets, I heard a loud rushing sound just behind me. I turned to see what it was. I was hit under by two feet of rushing muddy water and a whirlwind. I began running as hard and as fast as I could. Stopping to catch my breath, I found myself beside my car. I noticed a man along the passenger side, removing the fender. Walking to the other side, he ripped almost every part of the body and interior.

Furious, I demanded he get away from my car. Unshaken by my demands, he told me without reservation that the car was his and that I should get lost. More determined than ever, I told him I would not, because it was my car. I had the keys and the title that showed I was the rightful owner. Paying no attention, he continued to remove parts. Seeing he was not going to quit, I went inside the store to call the police.

There was a young guy by the telephone, but he was not using it. When I walked up and reached for the receiver, he said, "It will not do any good to call, because the guy outside does as he pleases. Stealing from anyone he wants." Then he said, "The guy is a bully and will continue to be so until someone shows his or her authority over him."

Looking out the window, I noticed a large group of people across the street in a wooded area. It looked as if they were having some type of party or parade. As I approached the crowd, I noticed a woman in a police uniform. I walked up to her and explained what the man was doing to my car. She informed me that they had been after him for a long time. They had been unable to catch him because people would not stand up to him. As long he could steal from them, he would.

At this point, I woke up. It was 7:30 a.m. I thought, *Why haven't they come in to weigh me?* Then it hit me. *Wow! What a dream! Boy, I'm going to have to get someone to interpret this dream just like King James did.* All of a sudden the Spirit of the Lord said, "No, Ron, you don't. I will tell you exactly what the dream meant.

"For a long time, Satan has tried to take you out. Out of God's will, out of living the Christian life, out of ministering to others, out of everything God has for your life. He and his demons have set traps along the way to cause your defeat and end. Tonight was no exception. Again, they [the demons] showed up, determined to wipe you out. They were on assignment straight from hell. When you awakened, you startled them. At the moment your eyes made contact with them, they could not come any closer. The light in your eye was too much for them. For the light they encountered, was the Light of God. Being covered by the blood of Jesus makes it impossible for them to destroy or take you out.

"In your dream the guy was stealing and robbing parts off your car. In reality, Satan does the same thing. He determines that everything we have or hope to have, including our life, is his. He will definitely take it from us unless we rise to the occasion and put him in his place.

"Once we come into the family of God, be assured, attacks from Satan do not stop. His primary job is to attack and accuse Christians. As we grow in the Lord, we will reach a level where we can recognize Satan's attacks and temptations. The most powerful tools we have against Satan are God's Word [the Bible] and prayer. As we stand up to him and walk in our righteousness—being a child of the Most High and washed in the blood of Jesus—he will back off. In God's Word, James 4:7 states, "Submit yourselves therefore to God, resist the devil and he flee from you." So there are two things in this Scripture we must do to have victory over the devil's attacks. First, *submit* to God, and second, *resist* the devil. Once we do these two things, we begin to see ourselves as overcomers. Each time, it becomes easier to put the devil in his place.

"The beauty of the mountain scene is a reminder that, even in the midst of destruction and calamity, we can still have peace and assurance that everything is going to be all right. Everything around us may be falling apart. Nothing going our way. Nowhere to turn. We may be at the point where we want to give up and die. Right where Satan wants us. That's where we have to be strong in the Lord. Call on His name, and believe that He is who He says he is. We must be willing to stand until victory comes.

"The part concerning the dogs trapped in the rushing waters—with you appearing with them, cutting through the floor—shows how Satan can deceive us. He is a master in making people believe that things are not as they truly are. Satan will use the closest things to us to deceive us and lead us astray. In doing so, we are often caught in a trap we cannot escape. Sadly, many have ended in perilous calamity and gone into eternity deceived. They believed they had made the right decision, only to find out that the results were fatal."

As I meditated on what the Spirit of God revealed to me, I started to weep with joy. I had come through so much. No matter how difficult things seem, we can always be assured, as long as we put our trust and hope in God, that we will forever come out on top.

From that day on, I didn't throw up. I did have a few more days when I gagged from taking breathing treatments. That soon was resolved by changes in my medication. I continued to trust God's Word and won the battle. After twenty-two days in the hospital I was discharged. I walked out of the hospital, removed my mask, and lifted my head and shouted, "Praise God." The feeling was truly incredible.

The weeks following my discharge, *Studio Plus became our permanent residence until we returned to North Carolina. Our favorite places to go were Kohl's, Target, Old Navy, and Culver's restaurant. * Studio Plus is a motel that offers a room that is a like an efficiency; includes a small kitchen,with dishes,sink, eating and sitting area.

Knowing we would be there, (in Madison), during Christmas, Shawnee's sister Lisa purchased us a small Christmas tree, decorations, and stockings to hang in the window. By the time Christmas arrived, our wall was covered with cards from family and friends. Though we were not home for Christmas, we still had a great celebration. On Christmas day, we awoke to a light dusting of snow. It's been a long time since we experienced snow on Christmas day. Though we missed our family back home, we got to spend the holiday with family in Wisconsin. On Christmas morning, we drove to Lancaster, an hour and half away, to spend the night with Lisa, Terry, and their sons, Steven and Derek. On Monday, December 26 (my fifty-third birthday), we drove to Lyndon Station to spend the day with Shawnee's mom and stepdad, John. Shawnee's brother Buster, her sister Jo, her husband, Darryl, and their daughters, Erica and Jacqlyn, were there also. We had a great day of food and visiting with family. Later in the evening, I was surprised when they brought out a birthday cake and sang "Happy Birthday" to me.

On our way back to Madison, we stopped in Baraboo to see Shawnee's brother Poncho and his wife, Jill. They have three sons. Only the youngest son, Reed, was there. Phillip and Spencer were with their mom. After a brief visit, we drove back to the apartment in Madison. We were exhausted after traveling about 240 miles that day and visiting with family in three different towns.

Starting the week of December 7th, the next three weeks, Shawnee and I remained in the studio apartment and made almost daily trips to the hospital for tests, X-rays, and clinic appointments. During that time, I entered a rehab program where I was able to rebuild strength in my arms, legs, and entire body. Tuesday, December 28 was our departure date to return home, and we were ecstatic about leaving. The day before, we went to the hospital for pulmonary lab tests and a bronchoscope (in which they scrape the lungs to check for rejection). On Tuesday afternoon, as we waited for the tests results, Shawnee finished packing the car.

The phone rang. Jumping to my feet, I answered the phone ready to hear, "You're free to go." But that wasn't the case. It was my transplant coordinator. "Don't leave. We need you to check in at the hospital; your bronch shows rejection." I almost fell to the floor. Anything would have been better than what I had just heard. Our hearts had been set on "good news" to set us "free" on the road to home. The only thing to do was to go to the hospital.

Once I was in my hospital room, the nurse came in and told us I was to receive medicine through IV that day and two more dosages over the next couple days. I knew this was for the best, and I was reminded from within that God was in control. Knowing that, I laid everything to rest and followed instructions. After all, what's another couple of days? We had been in the Madison area for three and half months.

Friday morning, December 31, I was released from the hospital and given permission to leave for home. This time was for real. As we made our way down the road toward the interstate, we were beside ourselves. We could hardly believe it. Shawnee was so ready to be home, she drove ten hours that day. We stopped about one hour north of Knoxville, Tennessee, we retired for the evening. The next morning, New Year's Day 2000, we had breakfast and drove three hours, arriving home shortly after the noon hour. The next morning, we got up and attended church. It was really nice to see all our friends and church family, and to say thank-you for all the support and prayers given on my and Shawnee's behalf. Our associate pastor welcomed us back home and asked if I would share part of my testimony. How God has blessed us not only with one lung, but both. I emphasized over and over how grateful I was that God saw fit to give me a second chance. He has done exceedingly great things for me, and I want to let the whole world know how great our Lord and Savior is.

During the next two weeks, Shawnee stayed home and got things set up for me. We had a lot of things to prepare before she returned to work. On Monday, January 17, Shawnee returned to work after being gone on family medical leave for four months. That first week was very hard on her. By the time she got home in the evening, she was exhausted. I tried to help as much as I could, but it wasn't much relief. Whenever possible, I tried to cook supper and pick up around the house. Though it was hard at times, we made out better than expected.

Four months after my transplant, healing was still at hand. Discipline was still very important. What I mean is, every day I had to remember to stay on schedule with my medications, breathing treatments, vitals, and exercises. When I got home, I was taking over fifty pills per day.

Each day I start out by taking my vital signs, weight, blood, and sugar count. I use my inhaler and then blow into a spirometer (an instrument that measures lung capacity). I have to repeat these procedures twice a day. This is a way of life. Anything less could cause a disaster. Along with my day-to-day recovering, I have to return to UW Hospital every three months for clinic appointments and tests for the next year. Then I'll have checkups every six months, and then yearly—unless rejection or other complications occur.

The first year of clinic appointments were gruesome. Our travel from Asheville to Madison was more than 925 miles one way. I believe we traveled to Madison six times in 2000. Also that year, Shawnee's brother Poncho and his wife, Jill, had a new baby girl, Lizzy. Receiving my transplant so close to her birth allowed me to bond with her precious life as a newborn. I felt such a connection just holding her. She showed me how precious life really is.

Closing Comments

———❧———

He brought me up also out of a

horrible pit, out of the miry clay,

and set my feet up on a rock,

and established my goings.

(Psalms 39:2)

God has taught me a lot over the past fifteen months. One thing is discipline. I really had to adjust my life like never before. I have always been the type to get up and go until I am exhausted. If I needed to skip a meal or put off something till later, I did. When dealing with situations concerning your health, you learn quickly that skipping a meal, forgetting to take medicine on time, or not exercising properly can seriously affect your way of living—or even kill you.

Another thing God has taught me is patience. There again, I've always been the type to be in a hurry. I can't wait to see the finished product. I can't stand to wait at traffic lights. (I'm sure I'm not the only one.) If you are all over the road or drive too slow, watch out for me. Forget following directions. I just want to hurry and get things done as quickly as possible—only to find out later that I needed that "extra" part to put it together correctly.

This is the way many Christians live: no instructions, no map, no focus, no purpose in mind. God is teaching me (He is still having to work overtime) to slow down, think things through, resting occasionally, and not expect everything to fall in place or be completed at once. It's hard when you've been used to working in hurry-up mode. But I'm learning. These things are more important to me now than ever before.

Shawnee and I also had the opportunity to see God manifest Himself in the lives of many people. During and after the transplant, several of the nurses' lives at UW hospital were gloriously changed as a result of what God did for Shawnee and me. I was able to share Jesus and His great love day after day. Some were set free from tobacco, and relationships were renewed and made stronger. Yet I truly feel that we both received much more from them than they did from us. A lot of things were accomplished for the glory of God. And I know that the changes in those lives (and the lives yet to be touched) were God-sent and will make a difference so long as those receiving the change heed what He has done for them.

Society needs more education on the importance of becoming an organ donor. I know that when we renew our driver's license, we're often asked if we would like to become a donor. Some do, some don't. If we could only see and understand that a life can be saved by the loss of another, we would all generously give our organs without reservation. So many lives are robbed of this most precious second chance because organs are not readily available. After receiving my lungs, I am more determined to spread the news about the importance of becoming an organ donor. The bumper sticker saying could not be truer: "Don't take your organs to Heaven; Heaven knows we need them here."

I am truly grateful for the technology in the world of science and medicine. God has given humankind the ability to create cures for so many sicknesses and diseases we face. As never before, I know that God renders healing according to our faith. If our faith leads us to trust God to bring healing through surgery, then I believe our healing will be administered that way. If we desire to trust God for supernatural healing, then I believe healing will come forth, so long as you believe and do not waver. In James 1:6, God tells us to "ask in faith, nothing wavering." How a person decides to receive healing depends on whether he or she trusts in surgery or in supernatural intervention. Either way, I believe it's like God told me: "All healing is of the Lord." That is what I believe. What you believe is totally up to you.

I would like to express my sincere thanks and gratitude to all those who stood by Shawnee and me during the times before, during, and after my lung transplant.

Thanks for the thousands of prayers offered on our behalf and for all the cards of encouragement and financial blessings. I am grateful for those who believed that God was with us. You'll never know how much it means to know that God's people are standing with you. Without prayer, I do not believe I would have been able to come through the transplant surgery like I did. Prayer does change things.

Above all, we give thanks and praise to the One who is worthy of our praise—our Lord Jesus Christ, in whom all blessings flow. Glory to God. God is great and greatly to be praised. I thank Him daily for the second chance at life He has given me. May I forever endeavor to do my best to please the God of heaven and earth—the One who not only created me but also died and rose again that I might have eternal salvation in Him. All He asks in return is that we confess our sins and trust Him to guide and direct us.

He has done exceedingly great things for me, and I wish to let the whole world know how great our Lord and Savior is. He did not have to give me new lungs, but He did. He did not have to give me a second chance, but He did. It was not He that made me live the life that I did. I chose to participate in a habit that was hazardous to my health.

Millions upon millions choose every day to sell themselves over to cravings (be it cigarettes, drugs, alcohol, or sex) that lead to destruction of the body. More times it destroys the soul, too, and has destroyed some spirits. God forbid that people would sell themselves over to addictions intended to destroy them. The Word of God reminds us that the thief (Satan) comes "to steal, kill and destroy." (John 10:10.)

God also tells us our bodies are the temple of God. I was an abuser of my own body. I was one of those who thought, *I'll quit whenever I choose to. I can lay cigarettes down any time I make my mind up.* That's what Satan wants us to believe. But it doesn't happen that way. The only way to quit any bad habit or addiction is deliverance by divine intervention. But you may say, "Wait a minute. I know of someone who quit cold turkey." That may be true; I've known of people that quit by walking away and never returned to their addiction. God is no respecter of persons. I believe that believers and nonbelievers can determine inside their hearts to give up a habit or addiction, and God will honor that wish, desire, or confession in various ways and on various timetables. Each and every one of us is uniquely made by God, and each of us responds differently in our own time.

What works for one may not work for another. My advice is, don't try to change your life by what someone else has experienced. Be sensitive to the voice of God, way down inside of your heart. Some would call this your gut feeling. By faith (the only way to please God), reach out and start applying a change in your everyday walk. Soon you will experience your life can have new meaning and purpose.

A month or so after that Sunday morning service, God spoke to us about assisting our friends' pastors, Wade and Gwen Hall, in a ministry that had been birthed in the wee hours of Saturday, November 13, 1999. They are the ones God woke early that morning to pray concerning my transplant.

In February 2000, our fellowship started holding Sunday-evening services in a meeting room a local motel. A couple of weeks later, we were at the pastor's home. Pastor Gwen was at her piano going over music for an upcoming service. As she played and sang, I soon found myself singing along with the others. Gwen commented, "Why, Ron, I didn't know you could sing."

In the weeks that followed, I began assisting in praise and worship. It wasn't long till a precious sister, Robin, encouraged me to sing a solo. I went to the bookstore and purchased a performance tape. After several weeks of practice and continued encouragement, I stood before the congregation and sang. Thank God I wasn't alone; Robin was there to back me up. Not long after, I purchased another tape, practiced it, and sang again.

Since that time, God has been so gracious to allow me to add more than thirty performance tapes to the music ministry. I give God all the glory and praise, for He and He alone has blessed me with the ability to sing. I thank Him and desire to continue in the path He leads me.

I received my new lungs three years ago. For the past week or so, I have had a cold or virus. It's one of the few times I have had a cough or sniffles in three years. My pulmonary doctors are quick to monitor my progress, should I come down with any symptoms. If an infection is left long, rejection could set in, and I could lose my lungs. God gives us wisdom, and we should apply it to our everyday walk.

A little over fifteen months after the transplant surgery, I decided to go along with a friend, Jim, to a sports show in neighboring Greensboro. Each day, I am to do breathing tests by blowing as hard as possible into a spirometer. The readings help determine whether my body is using the medicines required to maintain my transplanted lungs.

On Thursday, the first day after the sports show, I tested my breathing before breakfast. After entering the pretest information and doing three tests, I retrieved the results and recorded them just as I normally do. *Boy!* I thought, *these numbers are really down.* That evening, I decided to recheck. My results were worse than the other ones. I remarked to Jim, "If my numbers continue to spiral down, I may have to go home."

On Friday morning, again before breakfast, I tested and my results were down from the previous reading. I told Jim I had better have my wife come down the next morning to take me home. The weather that morning was cool but beautiful. The sun was bright, and there were hardly any clouds in the sky. The three-hour ride home was relaxing, yet I was really concerned that rejection might be taking place. That night, I had a good night's rest. The next morning, the test readings were really bad. We decided I had better call UW Hospital.

The receptionist on call that morning said she would have my coordinator return my call after referring with my transplant doctor. Within thirty minutes, we received a call requesting us to take the earliest flight possible to Madison. I found a flight with a departure time of 12:30 p.m., and we arrived in Madison just past four. A taxi took us directly to the hospital.

Immediately, hospital personnel began tests to determine my condition and a solution to stop the rejection. I had an IV in my arm and a high dosage of liquid prednisone to stabilize the rejection. Over the next couple of days, the prednisone was cut in half. We started making plans to return home, banking on the idea that the prednisone had done its job and everything was fine. But on Friday, my coordinator told me that they had been unable to determine what was causing my rejection, so we would have to stay several more days until the doctors could work out a solution. I was hoping we could make flight arrangements for our return home. Late Friday evening, my coordinator returned to inform us the doctors had decided to change my rejection medicines. The change would help my body accept the medicines better. But I would have to remain in the hospital to see if my body would accept the new medication.

Monday evening brought a sigh of relief as we received news that my body was responding nicely to the change of medicine. We were briefed on changes we needed to make and could fly out the following day. Again God had intervened and brought me through a situation that seemed hopeless.

Upon returning home, the pharmacist had to order the medicine, because it was not something they normally dispensed. Part of my rejection medicine was in pill form; the rest was an awful-tasting liquid that had to be dispensed from a syringe and mixed with orange juice. I hated getting up every morning to swallow that medicine, but I knew there was no way out of it. Every day I would pray, "God, please let them make this medicine in pill form." Guess what. Within about six months, the company came out with a coated pill. Praise God! God knew how much I hated that medicine. He answered my prayer. Hallelujah! God wants us to be happy even when taking medicine. What an awesome God we serve.

Over the last twenty-two months, I have been rejection free. My last couple visits to UW hospital did not require a bronch test, which is a relief. Every time I had a bronch, I got sick. There were times that I shook uncontrollably. After the first couple of experiences, the doctor prescribed two Tylenol to ward off the shakes. The sedation during the test is very mild, yet I hardly remember what takes place. Most of the time, I end up in recovery talking out of my head, making no sense at all. During one procedure, I said my wife hadn't come with me, but my daughter had. Another time I told the nurse she should come back to North Carolina. Boy, it's amazing what one will say when drugged up.

During my annual checkup in 2002, the doctor wanted me to see a specialist concerning the effects of medications on my kidneys. Upon returning home, I contacted Mountain Kidney Association for an appointment. In December, the doctor explained in detail my kidney functions, future risks, and preventive measures, and sent me for an outpatient kidney biopsy.

In January 2003, I returned to the kidney center for a follow-up. The doctor aid my kidney function was at only 30 percent of normal. He told me not to get alarmed, because I could live the rest of my live at that level. My kidney function would have to be closely monitored, and some of my medicines would have to be increased, decreased, or changed periodically to prevent further deterioration.

At present, my creatine levels associated with my lungs have been good and remain steady. Each time I return for blood labs, they check my kidney functions and creatine levels.

Over the years, God has impressed me to share my testimony and songs with other friends and strangers alike. I know God can use this ministry to touch people, set people free from addiction, heal those who need a healing, and give hope to those who desire an answer for their problems.

I understand God has a plan for each of our lives, and I know His love and mercy has been extended to me a second time, so I must share what He has done for me.

What you've read up to now has covered a five-year period: 1997 through 2003. Many things have transpired in my life since then. It is now July 2012. I have had many ups and downs, yet God is true to His Word. He has been with me all the way; He has never let me down. He has brought me through many battles and given me many more blessings. At times, Satan tries to derail me and throw some type sickness on me. But, thanks be to God, His Word always comes through. No matter what Satan sends our way, he is defeated.

Last month, I spent eight hours on a Saturday recording my first music CD. I am waiting to hear from the studio concerning final editing and approval. It has been a long coming, but I know God, has opened this door for me to have a tool to spread His message of love, healing, and deliverance to a hurting world.

Having this book published has been a dream and desire of mine for years. Soon after my transplant, I spent hours, weeks, and months writing details concerning my addiction to cigarettes, COPD, and emphysema. I want to inform everyone about the effects addiction can have on an individual.

My addiction happened to be cigarettes. Others are addicted to drugs, alcohol, lust—you name it. The end result is control—control over your life, emotions, esteem, and integrity. Addictions have ruined millions of lives. I'm here to tell you, you do not have to be one of the statistics.

There is a way you can be free from bondage and addiction. "The Way" is Jesus. His Word tells us He is "the Way, the Truth and the Life." Jesus died that we might have life and have it more abundantly. Just reach out to Him. He is close by and will answer your prayer.

God is continuing to open new opportunities for me to serve Him. I have been able to build a collection of over 185 songs for use in ministry. Each time the Lord opens a door to minister, He allows me to sing and minister under His anointing. Now, with the publication of my life experiences in book form, I have some tools by which God's love, grace, and glory can be shared.

My dream is to serve my Lord and Savior, Jesus Christ. To do my part. To lead others to a life free from sin, addiction, and despair.

"To God be the Glory, for the great things He has done." May God be exalted throughout the earth. His mercy endures forever.

About the Author

—————➤●◄—————

Ron Davis has always been an outgoing, knowledgeable, "fun to be with" type person. He is forever saying something that will cause you to come closer, to listen to what he has to say. It may funny, serious, or whatever, but never a dull moment. He is one of those persons you notice when he enters the room. He is never lost for words. He believes that everyone should be themselves and express their opinion without reservation. Everyone may not agree with your opinion or idea. If you hold on to your opinions or ideas without releasing them for others, might result in a great loss that would prove otherwise, useful to the entire world.

Thinking back years ago as a young business person, I introduced an idea that would utilize the industry that I represented. Everyone one of my superiors stated that I would not be able to pull it off. Never the less, I stood my ground, proceeded to prove them wrong. Months, later the main office noticed that my idea was working also saved time and freed up a lot of man hours, for all those working in the field.

Today, the idea I introduced, has become standard practice in the newspaper industry. I suggest to anyone that might have an idea, thought or suggestion. Do not keep it hidden inside. Release it and get it out. You never know what might come forth from just a thought. Our universe and way of life today is a result of an idea or thought someone released.

I live in the beautiful smoky mountains, of Western North Carolina, Asheville, about one hundred miles west of Charlotte. I am retired and travel area churches, and attend special events sharing the good news of a bilateral lung transplant and singing gospel music with the lungs God blessed me with.